PRACTICAL ESCRIMA KNIFE DEFENSE

FILIPINO MARTIAL ARTS KNIFE DEFENSE TRAINING

SAM FURY

Illustrated by
GIACOMO PILATO

WARNINGS AND DISCLAIMERS

The information in this publication is made public for reference only.

Neither the author, publisher, nor anyone else involved in the production of this publication is responsible for how the reader uses the information or the result of his/her actions.

CONTENTS

THANKS FOR YOUR PURCHASE

Did you know you can get FREE chapters of any SF Nonfiction Book you want?

https://offers.SFNonfictionBooks.com/Free-Chapters

You will also be among the first to know of FREE review copies, discount offers, bonus content, and more.

Go to:

https://offers.SFNonfictionBooks.com/Free-Chapters

Thanks again for your support.

INTRODUCTION

In this self-defense training manual, Sam Fury puts Vortex Control Self-Defense lessons learned in the Philippines onto paper.

Vortex Control Self-Defense is a unique fighting system created by Peter Sunbye. To create this system of self-defense, Peter traveled for 20+ years, searching for "lost" self-defense techniques.

He combined a number of martial arts, including GM Lawrence Lee's Tong Kune Do kung fu, Wing Chun, Balintawak Arnis Escrima, and Panatukan to create a highly effective and relatively easy to learn self-defense system. Once the basics are learned, Vortex Control Self-Defense can be applied effectively by almost anyone, regardless of their dexterity, strength, or fitness level.

This volume covers knife defense. Knife defense is the ability to defend yourself against an attacker who has a knife, though the techniques used can be applied to many other weapon attacks.

Knife fighting is extremely dangerous. In real life, it must be avoided at all costs. Never expect to go into a knife fight and come out unharmed. Even if you "win," you'll probably get cut, or worse. Be sure to use a training knife when practicing the techniques described here.

This publication has been written under the approval of Peter Sunbye.

What follows is an excerpt from www.VortexControlDefence.com.

Some small edits have been made for ease of reading, but the meaning is unaltered.

∾

There is an ongoing debate about the efficiency and real usability of different defenses against knives and sharp objects. There are also different opinions on the focus of the defense. Our system (Vortex Control Self-Defense, or VCSD) attacks the attacker.

The "block/grab" knife defense system by GM Larry Alquezar is the foundation of our system. It has been shown to be very effective against other objects. This foundation is instilled into the practitioner through flow drills, retention drills, and extension into realistic use.

~

EXPLANATION OF TERMS

A few terms are used throughout this book to help describe the flow of movement.

Lead/Rear Side

Your lead side is whichever side of your body is forward-most and your rear side is whichever side of your body is rear-most. For example, if you're in a right-foot-forward stance, then your right side is your lead side, and your left side is your rear side.

Inside/Outside of Your Opponent's Guard

When your opponent's guard is up, you can place your arm either inside or outside of it.

Being inside your opponent's guard means that your limb is in between his limbs, closer to his center. Your arm is sandwiched by his.

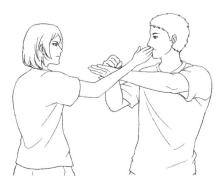

Being outside your opponent's guard means your opponent's limbs are both to either the left or right of your limb.

The pictures demonstrate being inside/outside of your opponent's guard with your arms, but it also applies to your legs. That is, you need to step to the outside of your opponent's guard in order to get behind him.

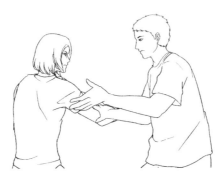

Just as you can be inside or outside your opponent's guard, he can be inside/outside yours.

Guarding Your Opponent's Limb

The expression "to guard your opponent's limb" means to put your limb close or on his limb so that you can't be struck by it. It is a pre-emptive defensive maneuver that may also be referred to as "covering your opponent's limb."

Throughout this book, the word "limb" is replaced as appropriate. For example, in the previous picture the man is using his right hand to guard/cover the woman's right elbow.

PRINCIPLES OF SELF-DEFENSE

The following principles are the core of Vortex Control Self-Defense. Although explained in reference to hand-to-hand combat, they are also applicable to weaponry.

Without these principles, the rest of this book is just a bunch of techniques that you can mimic. With them, the techniques in this book become a collection of examples of how the principles can be applied. You can then replicate techniques and/or create customized to ones.

The Vortex Control Self-Defense principles are all of equal importance, and are presented here in alphabetical order.

Constant Barrage

In Vortex Control Self-Defense there, you are constantly slapping, twisting, pulling, and pushing your opponent. This serves at least one (and usually several, if not all) of the following purposes:

- It confuses and disorients your opponent.
- It often lets you move your opponent one way while striking from the opposite direction. This increases the force of your strike.
- The movements in themselves bring a certain degree of discomfort and pain.
- It lets you place your opponent in the ideal position for your next move.

This also makes use of Newton's first law of motion, which states that:

> "An object at rest stays at rest, and an object in motion stays in motion with the same speed and in the same direction unless acted upon by an unbalanced force."

In reference to your movement, this means that it's better for you to keep moving once you're in motion. This is because it takes more energy to stop and restart than it does to continue an existing motion. In addition, the continued motion will be faster and therefore more powerful than if you were to start from inertia.

Counters

In martial arts, a counter is an attack made in response to your opponent's attack. It is about being proactive.

There is always a counter to your opponent's move, and there is a counter to your counter, and a counter to that counter. It can go on forever. The victor will be whoever has the foresight and/or intuition to out-counter their opponent.

Close combat is a game of chess. Fast chess. Instinctive chess.

Note: The closer you get to your opponent, the fewer opportunities there are for counters. You can use this to your advantage by first closing distance while gaining an advantageous position, and then finishing the fight before your opponent recovers.

Grounding

Grounding yourself means being in solid contact with the ground.

When you're grounded, you have more stability, and can therefore generate more powerful attacks. Power in strikes comes up from the ground. This is a well-known concept in the world of martial arts.

A simple exercise you can do to get the feeling of grounding is to pretend that you're drilling your body into the ground.

The act of grounding can also be used to increase damage by letting gravity do the work. To get the feeling of using grounding in this manner, lift both your legs off the ground without jumping. Just let gravity do its thing.

Fulcrums

Body mechanics, paired with physics, play a big part in the efficiency of Vortex Control Self-Defense. By using parts of your body as fulcrums, you can gain more leverage, apply locks, break limbs, etc.

One-Handed Fighting

Both arms are used in the demonstrations in this book, but the un-armed portion of Vortex Control Self-Defense is developed so that most of the techniques can be done one-handed. This becomes extremely useful in real-life scenarios, such as when you are holding something you can't drop, like a baby, or when your arm gets injured. Once you have a good grasp of the techniques, you should train to do them with one hand. Just don't use your rear hand.

Power Angles

This is another principle based on physics and body mechanics.

There are certain angles that create the strongest frames. Your limbs should never be below 120° or above 160°.

120° is best for defense. Any smaller of an angle, and your arm will easily collapse when it's pushed towards you.

160° is best for attack. Any larger of an angle, and your arm can be easily pushed to the side. Holding it at an angle greater than 160° will also make it more susceptible to being captured—by being placed in a lock, for example.

As a rule, keep your limb at 120°. When you strike, extend it to 160° and then let your body push through. This combines power angles with grounding. Add in spring-loading and aim for the spine and you have the ideal the Vortex Control Self-Defense strike.

Spine Center

The Spine Center principle is based on the centerline theory, which is common in many martial arts, including Wing Chun. To explain the concept, here is an excerpt from the book *Basic Wing Chun Training* by Sam Fury:

www.SFNonfictionBooks.com/Basic-Wing-Chun-Training

Your centerline is an imaginary line drawn vertically down the center of your body. All the vital organs are located near the center of the body. Keep it away from your opponent by angling it away from him/her.

Controlling the position of your centerline in relation to your opponent's is done with footwork. Understanding the centerline will allow you to instinctively know where your opponent is.

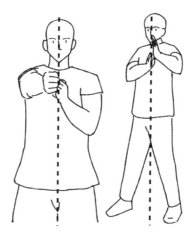

Your central line (different from your centerline) is drawn from your angled center to your opponent.

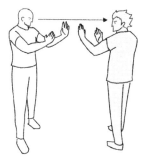

Offensively, you generate the most power when punching out from your center, since you can incorporate your whole body and hips.

When you're attacking in a straight line, your centerline should face away from your opponent, while your central line faces his/her center.

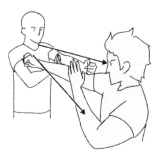

With hook punches and other circular attacks, the center- and central lines merge.

There are three main guidelines for the centerline.

- The one who controls the centerline will control the fight.
- Protect and maintain your own centerline while you control and exploit your opponent's.
- Control the centerline by occupying it.

In Vortex Control Self-Defense, instead of putting your offensive focus on your opponent's centerline as described above, focus on his spine. Doing so makes the idea of striking through your target more intuitive. An added advantage is that his spine can be affected by the many jerks, twists, etc. that are commonly used in Vortex Control Self-Defense.

Spring-Loading

Yet another principle based on the combination of body mechanics and physics is spring-loading.

The basic premise is that your muscles can be pushed in like a spring. These springs are then released in strikes, increasing speed and therefore power.

Speed in strikes is not just about how fast you reach the target. You must also be quick to recover. Recovery is the process of reloading the spring, which you can then send out again. In your arm, your triceps are the spring forward and your biceps are the spring back. Alternating spring-loading your arms allows you to make multiple strikes in very quick succession.

You can and should also spring-load your legs.

It's important to remain relaxed. The spring is loaded and released, but never tensed so much that it slows you down.

Taking Space

Always crowd your opponent. Get in his space and claim it. Constantly push him back, and don't let up. This will unbalance him both mentally and physically.

Following the Thank You Principle

Take whatever your opponent gives you and use it to your advantage. If he applies pressure in a particular direction, flow with it. Redirect it if needed, but don't directly oppose it.

Those that want to become really good at this are encouraged to practice Chi Sao. Although live instruction is always preferred, the book *How to do Chi Sao* by Sam Fury is highly recommended.

www.SFNonfictionBooks.com/Chi-Sao

Another use of the thank you principle is to always take something back. For example, when retracting your limb from a strike, grab your opponent's arm or nose-ring.

Vibrating

In Vortex Control Self-Defense, the principle of vibrating is used to enhance the effectiveness of movement. It can be applied in many situations, such as when you're increasing the force in locks, making repetitive strikes, escaping holds, etc.

The following examples offer safe demonstrations of the effectiveness of vibrating:

The first example is a shirt-grab escape. Say an attacker grabs you by the shirt-front. Reach over his arms and grab his right wrist. At the same time, use your left hand to grab the same arm.

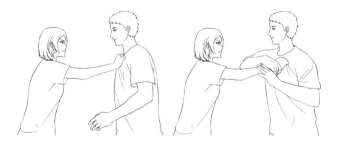

To release your opponent's grip, twist your body to your right using a waterfall motion.

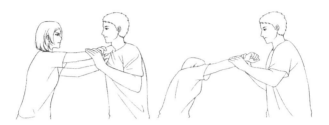

This move itself is a common and effective self-defense technique, but when your attacker is much stronger than you, it may not work. Increase its effectiveness by vibrating.

As you twist your body, make small, fast, jerking movements. Concentrate these movements into your twisting motion, especially where your opponent is gripping you.

The next example is a rear bear hug escape. Say an attacker puts you in a rear bear hug with your arms pinned. A common way to get out of this is with rear elbows, but if your opponent's grip is too tight, you won't have the room to do this. Vibrate your body to create space.

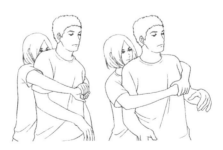

As soon as you have even just enough room, rear elbow left and then right. Finally, drop your body weight and ground yourself to break your opponent's grip.

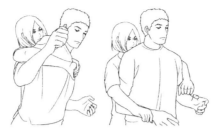

Vortex

By using the motion of a vortex (like water going down a sinkhole) you can easily break through your opponent's defense. For example, if your opponent is pushing your hand in a certain direction, you can use a vortex motion to move under and around it. This is actually the basis of the curve entry.

Another way to use the vortex is if your opponent grabs your arm. A fast vortex motion will most likely free you from his grip while you counter-strike in the same motion. In most cases, you'll want to vortex towards your opponent's spine.

Warfare Strategy

The strategy for attack in Vortex Control Self-Defense mimics that of warfare.

Intelligence. First, you must gather intelligence so you can make the right decision regarding your enemy. In warfare, this is done through methods such as espionage. In self-defense, it's better understood as "sizing up" your opponent.

Within a few seconds of studying your enemy, you can determine any weaknesses he has (such as obvious injuries), sense his fear (or lack thereof), assess his ability (speed, strength, skill), etc. You can also assess your surroundings and identify possible escape routes, available weapons, etc.

Bombs. After your initial assessment, assuming you feel that fighting is necessary, attack with bombs. The military uses planes and mortars. In Vortex Control Self-Defense, we use bomb-kicks.

Infantry. Finally, once the bombs have done their job, the infantry is sent in. This translates to the use of entry techniques and the fighting formula.

Waterfall

The analogy of water going over the edge of a waterfall is often used to explain how to perform certain movements used in the techniques. The free-fall of water is also akin to grounding. Combing the three actions of waterfall, grounding, and vortex is extremely powerful.

Weaponizing

The principle of weaponizing means to make as many of your movements as much like attacks as possible, even if they are primarily defensive or neutral. Here are some examples:

- Instead of just placing your foot down after a kick, stomp your opponent's knee or foot.
- When defending against an incoming strike, don't just block it. Instead, block it in a way that hurts your opponent as well. Punch his arm (a stop-hit), for example.
- Your intention may be to apply a lock, but you can make various strikes in the process.
- After hitting your opponent, hit him again while retracting your limb.

Yin and Yang

The well-known Chinese Taoism concept of yin and yang is also applied in Vortex Control Self-Defense, where yin is "soft" and yang is "hard."

Soft does not equal weak, and it is the combination of soft and hard, fast and slow, light and heavy (grounded), etc. that will make your techniques work together.

Here are some examples to demonstrate the use of yin and yang in the context of Vortex Control Self-Defense. These are just a few examples of a concept that applies to everything in the universe.

- Tai Chi is very yin (slow and soft) in practice, and to the layman it may seem useless for combat, but if you speed the movements up to become yang (hard and fast), they can be devastating.
- In training, it's useful to use more yin and less yang. Doing things slowly (yin) first allows your mind and body to "soak in" the lessons. If you go straight to yang, not only will you learn poor technique, but your chances of injury while training will also be much higher.
- When an opponent strikes, you can receive his attack using yin, going with the flow of his motion. You may also defend against it using yang, attacking your opponent's limb as he strikes. A third option is to use a combination of yin and yang, where you receive the attack by flowing with it and then redirect the energy to counterattack.
- When you're using your hand to meet an attack, if your fingers face forward, it is considered yin. If your fingers face up, it's Yang. When your fingers are up, the hard, bony part of your hand is exposed, but when your fingers are forward it's not.

ATTACK

In the demonstrations in this book, the attacker will always hold the knife in his right hand. When the description refers to a left attack, it means one in which the strike comes in on an angle from the attacker's left. The knife is still held in his right hand.

Note: The method of attack used in this book is intended to help you practice defense. For more effective knife attack methods, please refer to the bonus chapters.

Straight Thrust

A straight thrust is when an attacker strikes into your torso from waist height. It's always done using a forward grip.

Downward Stab

As its name suggests, the downward stab is an attack that comes in on a downward motion. It's always done using a reverse grip.

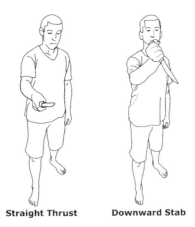

Straight Thrust   **Downward Stab**

DEFENSE

Every defense begins with the block/grab technique. This allows you to have two hands on your attacker's one, and is important because it gives you better control of his knife-wielding hand.

Unfortunately, using the block/grab technique ties up both your hands. This makes you vulnerable to being hit by your attacker's other hand, especially if you're slow to apply a disarm.

However, being hit is better than being stabbed, which (arguably) makes the block/grab a safer technique to use than others.

Unless otherwise stated, your grabbing hand is closer to your opponent's hand than your blocking hand is. You block on your opponent's lower forearm, but grab at his wrist.

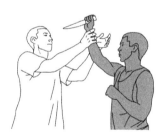

Blocks

There are two main types of blocks for knife defense: the chop and Bong Sau. How these blocks are applied depends on the situation, as well as on what works best for you.

To do the chop, use your forearm to chop down on your attacker's arm. Do it hard and aim for his upper forearm, since there is a cluster of nerves there. Often, this blow on its own will be enough to cause your attacker to drop his knife.

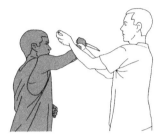

Bong Sau is taken from Wing Chun, but its application is modified depending on the situation. The images offer the best interpretation.

What follows is another excerpt *Basic Wing Chun Training* by Sam Fury.

Bong Sau (wing arm) is a defensive technique unique to Wing Chun. It's used to divert a punch by creating an angle of deflection.

Begin in the half squat position, with your hands up. In one movement, turn your hand down and your elbow up. As you do so, turn your waist and tilt your body so your feet are in a fighting stance. Your waist should do the work, not your arm.

Keep your arm in line. You other hand is a guard hand in case your opponent's strike passes through. This is Bong Sau.

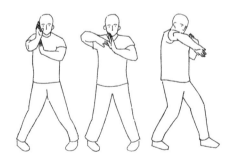

Turn slightly back and bring your hand back to the center.

Switch hand positions so your other hand becomes your lead. Shift your weight to match your new position and then do Bong Sau on your other side.

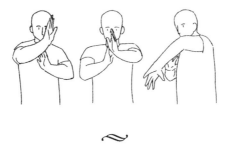

Grips

There are two types of grips.

An underhand grip is when your palm faces up or to the outside of your opponent's guard.

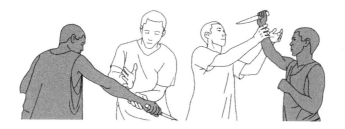

An overhand grip is when your palm faces down or to the inside of your opponent's guard.

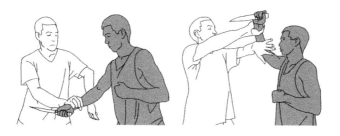

Making a Tap

In many of the disarms, once you've applied the block/grab technique, the next step is to "make a tap."

The term "making a tap" refers to the act of bending your opponent's wrist so his hand is at a 90° angle to his forearm. Doing this makes it easier to control his hand, twist his wrist, and therefore disarm him. A tap can be made at almost any of your opponent's joints. This makes it easier to apply locks.

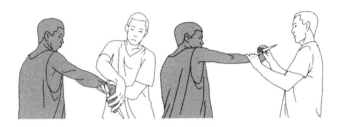

Grabbing Your Opponent's Hand

Unless otherwise stated, grabbing your opponent's hand means grabbing the fleshy part underneath his thumb. This helps loosen the grip your opponent has on his knife so you can take it.

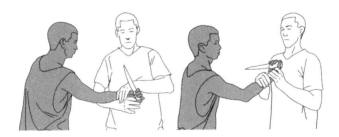

Grabbing the Knife

In many of the disarms, you're required to grab the knife in order to disarm your opponent. You need to do so in such a way that you do not cut yourself.

Grabbing the handle is the best way, but this won't be possible most of the time because your opponent will be gripping the handle. The next best option is to grab the blade from the blunt side. This assumes it is a single-edged knife.

The last option is to grip the blade between your fingertips and your palm in such a way that the sharp edge does not touch you.

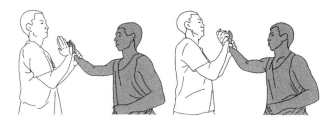

Aim to grab as much of the handle as possible when doing this, to minimize injury.

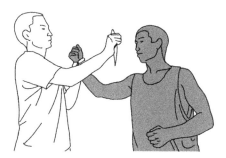

Taking the Knife

In most cases, you'll pull the knife towards your opponent's thumb and pry it out of his hand. This will take advantage of the weakest point in his grip.

KNIFE STEPPING DRILLS

These simple drills ingrain the foot to step in with in your muscle memory.

Knife Attack Stepping Drill

In a knife attack, step in using the foot on the same side as your knife strike is coming from.

The same side is not necessarily the same hand. In other words, just because you're holding the knife in your right hand doesn't mean the knife is coming in from the right-hand side.

Stand with your feet shoulder-width apart. This is the neutral position. Hold the knife in your right hand near your right shoulder, with a reverse grip.

At the same time, step in with your right foot as you stab down with your right hand. Your hand and foot should move at the same time, but your hand should hit your target before your foot lands.

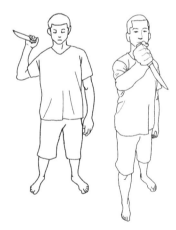

Step back to your original position with your right foot. As you do, bring your right hand to your left shoulder.

Step in with your left foot as you stab down from your left shoulder with your right hand.

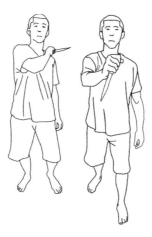

Return to the starting position and repeat the previous movements for a few minutes. When you're ready, change to a forward grip and hold the knife in your right hand near your right hip. Place your feet in the neutral position.

Step forward with your right leg and stab at the same time.

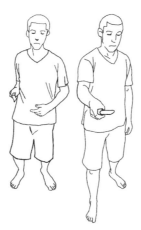

Step back into the neutral position as you bring your right hand back to the left side of your body. As you pull your hand back, rotate it so your palm faces up. This allows you to keep your knife pointed towards your opponent.

Step forward with your left foot and stab at the same time.

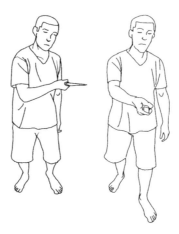

Return to your starting position and repeat the drill for a few minutes.

You can also go straight from the first part of the drill into the second. That is, you can do a right downward stab, left downward stab, right straight thrust, and left straight thrust.

Knife Defense Stepping Drill

In knife defense, it's best to step in using the foot that's opposite the side the knife attack is coming in on. If you step in with your left foot, block with your left hand and grab with your right, and vice versa.

The following drill focuses on stepping and blocking using the same hand.

Start in the neutral position, hands empty.

Step forward with your right foot and bring your right hand down to chop your imaginary opponent's forearm using a similar action as in the downward stab.

Use power angles (between 120° and 160°) at your elbow and wrist, with your fingers pointing towards your opponent.

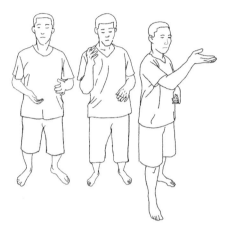

Return to the neutral position and then do the movement using your left side.

Next, do the same thing using Bong Sau.

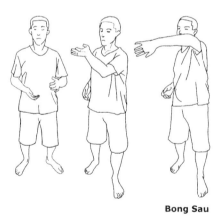

Bong Sau

The attack and defense drills can be practiced at the same time if you have a partner. One person attacks and the other defends.

The explanations of the drills shown above use simple angles and minimal body movement. This is for ease of explanation, but it's also a good place to start in practice.

In reality, attack and defense can be done on any angle, including curved hooking motions. You will need to bend your body depending on the situation.

Related Chapters:

- Attack
- Defense

GROUP A

Group A knife-defense techniques have the aim of taking the knife away from your attacker, and they all follow a similar pattern:

1. Block/grab.
2. Hand/thumb grab.
3. Create a "tap" (or twist the limb).
4. Disarm your opponent.

A1

Your opponent attacks with a right downward stab. Step in and block with your right using Bong Sau. Almost simultaneously, grab your opponent's wrist using an underhand grip.

Without losing contact with your opponent's arm, use your right hand to grab his right hand. Grab as much of his thumb as much as you can.

As you do this, turn your body so you are facing to your left.

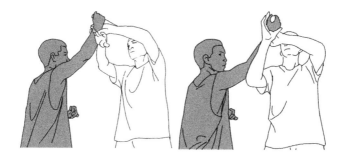

Bring your opponent's arm hard against your torso, at about the height of your solar plexus. If you haven't already, get a good grip on his thumb with your right hand.

Use your left hand to pry the knife out of your opponent's grip.

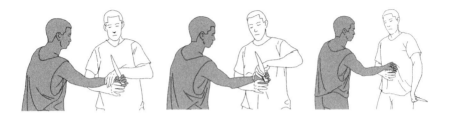

A2

Your opponent attacks with a left downward stab. Block with your left, using a chop. Grab your opponent's wrist with your right, using an underhand grip.

Use your left hand to grab your opponent's hand. Grab as much of his thumb as you can.

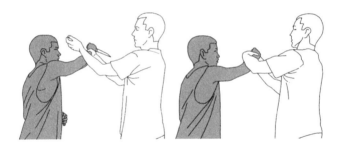

As you turn to your left, draw your elbows in to your body and bring your opponent's hand close to your chest.

Use your right hand to grab the knife and pry it out of your opponent's hand.

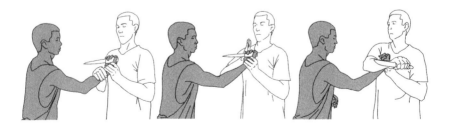

A3

Your opponent attacks with a right straight thrust. Defend with a right chop and left underhand grab. Use your left hand to grab your opponent's hand and bend his wrist down.

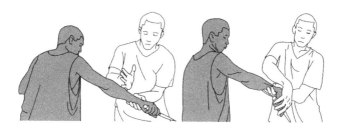

Without letting go of your hands, turn to your right so you're facing your opponent. This untwists you and leaves your opponent's elbow and hand facing up. Pry the knife toward your opponent to disarm him.

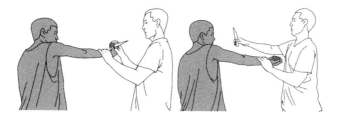

A4

Your opponent attacks with a left straight thrust. Chop block with your left and use an underhand grip with your right.

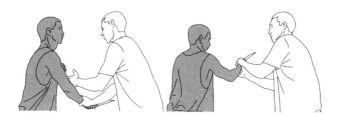

Use your left hand to grab your opponent's thumb, and then bring his hand up vertically.

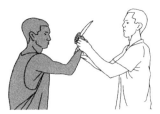

Bend your opponent's hand to the outside of his guard to perform a wrist lock, and then use your left hand to pry the knife out.

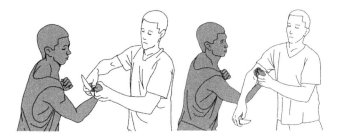

GROUP B

Group B techniques are used to inflict pain on your opponent.

The pattern is:

1. Block/grab.
2. Trap your opponent's hand.
3. Induce pain.
4. Disarm your opponent.

B1

Your opponent attacks with a right downward stab. Defend with a right Bong Sau and left underhand grab.

Without losing contact with your opponent's arm, use your right hand to grab his right hand so that he cannot let go of the knife.

As you do this, turn your body so you are facing to your left.

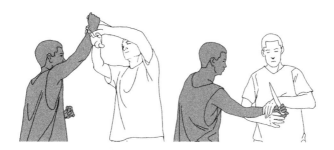

Bring your opponent's arm hard against your torso at about the height of your solar plexus.

Lean forward slightly to apply pressure and cause pain.

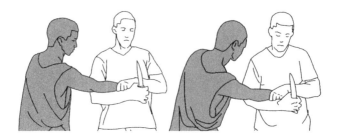

Release the pressure and then turn to face your opponent, while keeping hold of his arm.

Make the same downward motion to produce pain again, and then take the knife from your opponent.

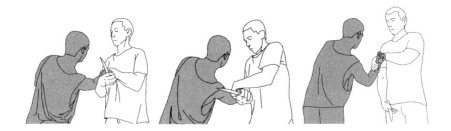

B2

B2 is basically the same as B1 apart from the block-and-grab combination used. In the following demonstration, it's shown from the opposite side to give you the benefit of a different view.

Your opponent attacks with a left downward stab. Defend with a left Bong Sau and right overhand grab.

Without losing contact with your opponent's arm, use your left hand to grab his right hand. Grab your opponent's hand so that he cannot let go of the knife. As you do this, turn your body so you're facing to your right.

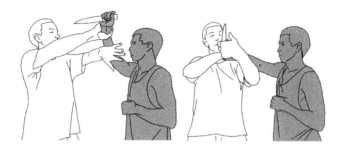

Bring your opponent's arm hard against your torso at about the height of your solar plexus.

Lean forward slightly to apply pressure and cause pain.

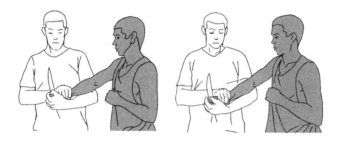

Release the pressure and then turn to face your opponent, while keeping hold of his arm.

Make the same downward motion to produce pain again, and then take the knife from your opponent.

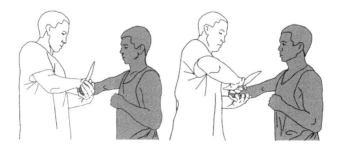

B3

Your opponent attacks with a right straight thrust. Defend using a right chop and a left overhand grab.

Bring your right arm underneath your left arm. The picture is exaggerated for demonstration purposes. You will probably not need to put your hand so close to your armpit.

Use your arm as a guide as you chop the back of your opponent's right hand. The purpose of this is to bend his wrist down.

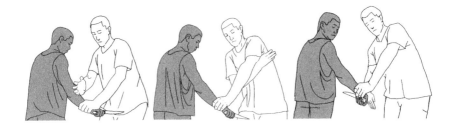

Bend your opponent's arm up and toward him. As you do this, change the grip of your right hand so that your palm is on the back of your opponent's hand.

Apply pressure on your opponent's wrist (toward the outside of his guard) to cause pain, and then disarm him.

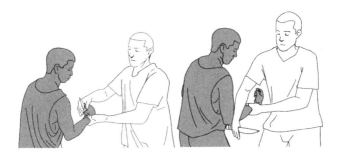

B4

Your opponent attacks with a left straight thrust. Defend using a left chop and right overhand grip.

Bring your left arm underneath your right arm, and then chop down on the back of your opponent's right hand.

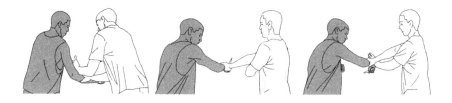

Guide your opponent's right hand to your left. Keep his arm straight. As you do this, grab his wrist with your left hand using an underhand grip. Continue the motion until his elbow faces up.

Shift your left hand from your opponent's wrist to the back of his hand.

Apply pressure to his wrist to cause pain, and then take the knife.

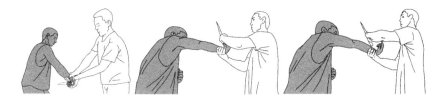

GROUP C

The techniques in group C cause the knife hand to cross from one side of your body to the other. The pattern used is:

1. Block/grab.
2. Disarm.

C1

Your opponent strikes with a right downward stab. As you move to the outside of his guard defend with a left Bong Sau and a right overhand grip. Curve your left arm over your opponent's right arm.

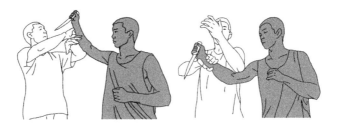

At the right moment, push your elbow down just above the crook of your opponent's elbow and grab the knife.

Pry the knife out of your opponent's hand, pulling to the outside of his guard.

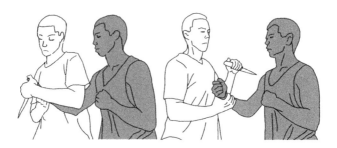

C2

Your opponent attacks with a left downward stab. Defend with a left chop and a right underhand grab.

Bend your opponent's right arm by applying downward pressure to the crook of his elbow with your left hand.

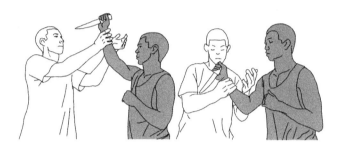

Grab the knife and pry it out of your opponent's hand, pulling toward the outside of his guard.

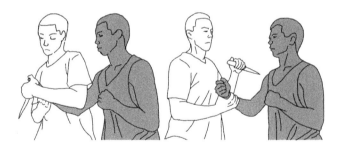

C3

Your opponent attacks with a right straight thrust. Defend with a right chop and a left overhand grab.

Bring your opponent's hand between your two bodies and to your right side.

As you do this, take an overhand grip on your opponent's right wrist with your right hand. Bring your left arm underneath it, perpendicular to his right arm.

The crook of your elbow should be underneath your opponent's elbow. Apply quick pressure by pulling back on his wrist while pushing on his elbow with your left upper arm.

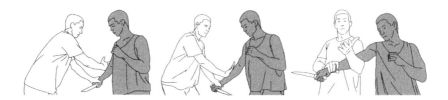

If your opponent hasn't dropped the knife yet, use your left hand to grip it from the top. Pull the knife towards your opponent and out of his grip.

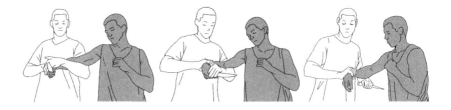

C4

Your opponent attacks with a left straight thrust. Defend using a left chop and right overhand grip.

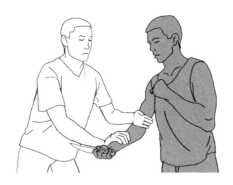

Curl your left arm underneath your opponent's right arm so it is perpendicular to it.

The crook of your elbow should be underneath your opponent's elbow. Apply quick pressure by pulling back on his wrist while pushing on his elbow with your left upper arm.

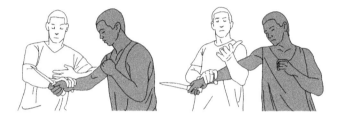

If your opponent hasn't dropped the knife yet, use your left hand to grip it from the top.

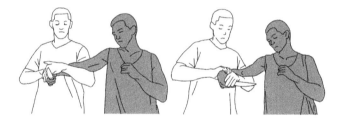

Pull the knife towards your opponent and out of his grip.

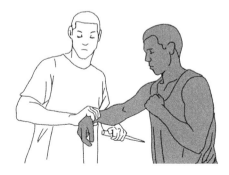

GROUP D

Group D techniques are ones you can do no matter which foot you use to step in first.

D1

Your opponent attacks with a right downward stab. Defend using a right Bong Sau and left overhand grip.

Place the edge of your right hand along the dull side of his blade.

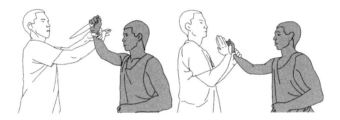

Pull the knife out toward your opponent.

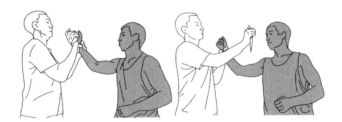

D2

Your opponent attacks with a left downward stab. Defend in the same way as D1, using a right Bong Sau and left overhand grip.

Place the edge of your right hand along the dull side of his blade.

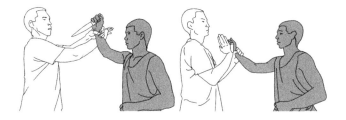

Pull the knife out toward your opponent.

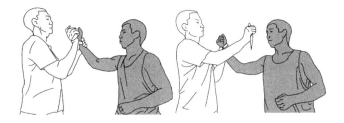

D3 (A)

Your opponent attacks with a right straight thrust. Defend with a left chop and right overhand grip, and then take an overhand grip with your left hand as well.

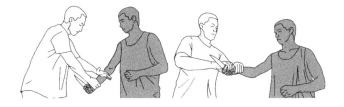

Use your right hand to apply pressure to your opponent's wrist. Release the pressure and then pry the knife out of your opponent's hand, pulling it toward him.

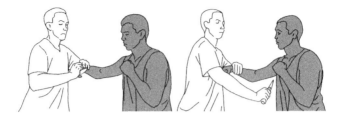

D3 (B)

Your opponent attacks with a right straight thrust. Defend with a right chop and left overhand grip.

Use your right hand to take an overhand grip on your opponent's arm.

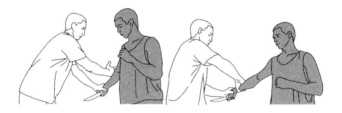

Twist your opponent's arm clockwise, so that his elbow faces up. Use you left hand to pry the knife out of your opponent's hand.

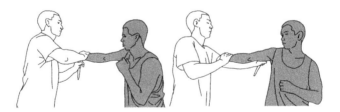

D4 (A)

Your opponent attacks with a left straight thrust. Defend using a right chop and left underhand grip. Adopt an overhand grip on your opponent's wrist with your right hand.

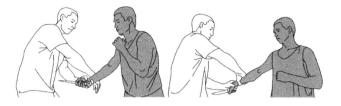

Twist your opponent's arm clockwise, so that his elbow faces up. Use your left hand to pry the knife out of your opponent's hand.

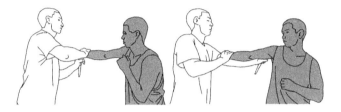

D4 (B)

Your opponent attacks with a left straight thrust. Defend using a left chop and right overhand grip.

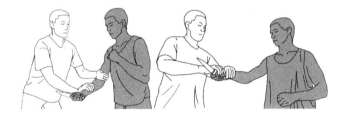

Adopt an overhand grip on your opponent's wrist with your left hand. Use your right hand to apply pressure to your opponent's wrist. Release the pressure and then pry the knife out of your opponent's hand, pulling it toward him.

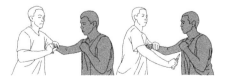

BREAKS

A break is when you break your opponent's limb. Each group of techniques demonstrated here also has a subset of break techniques.

A1 Break

Your opponent attacks with a right overhand stab. Defend with a right Bong Sau and a left underhand grab. Hold tight with your left hand and use your left forearm to attack your opponent's ribs.

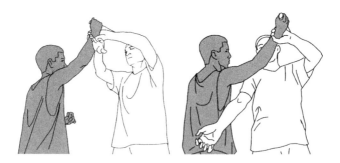

With the underside of your right arm facing up, strike upwards at your opponent's right elbow. At the same time, bring your opponent's right arm down with your left hand to apply an arm break. Use your right hand to grab your opponent's right hand/thumb.

Turn your body to your left, putting your back towards your opponent as you bring his right elbow over your shoulder. Apply pressure downwards to perform a second arm break.

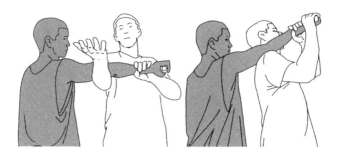

A2 Break

Your opponent attacks with a left downward stab. Use a left chop and a right overhand grip to defend.

Simultaneously use your right hand to twist your opponent's right hand and let your left forearm fall on your opponent's arm in a waterfall action (see the Principles of Self-Defense chapter). This will twist his elbow to face up and straighten his arm out at the same time.

Apply downward pressure to your opponent's elbow.

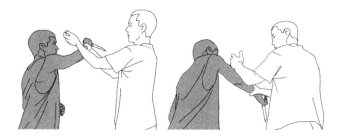

A3 Break

Your opponent attacks with a right straight stab. Defend using a right chop and a left overhand grab.

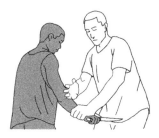

Step back with your right foot as you bring your opponent's right hand across your body. As you do this, adopt an overhand grip with your right hand.

Step in with your left leg and use your left forearm to strike/apply pressure on your opponent's right elbow.

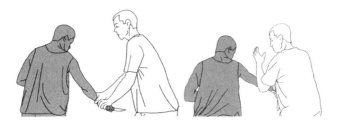

A4 Break

Your opponent attacks with a left straight thrust. Use a left chop and a right overhand grab to defend.

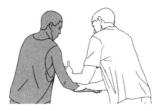

Pull your opponent's arm back and across your body to straighten it out. At the same time, bring your left arm back to create some space between it (your left arm) and your opponent's right arm.

Use your left forearm to strike/apply pressure on your opponent's right elbow.

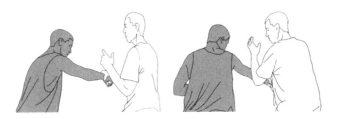

B1 Break

All B breaks use an overhand grip and the same arm-break technique.

Your opponent attacks with a right downward stab. Defend with a left Bong Sau and a right overhand grab.

Guide your opponent's right arm down as you shift your body to the outside of his guard.

As your opponent's right arm comes down, bring your right hand up on the inside of his guard. The intention is to grab your opponent's hand so he cannot let go of the knife.

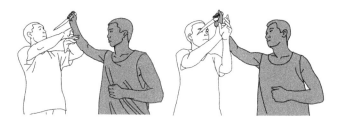

Continue to guide your opponent's arm down until it's horizontal and tight across your body. Your opponent's arm should sit snugly in the crook of your elbow.

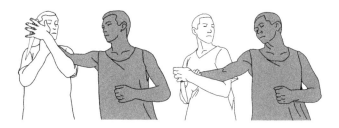

Apply the break by pulling your opponent's hand towards you while using your left upper arm to apply opposing pressure on his elbow.

B2 Break

Your opponent attacks with a left downward stab. Defend with a left chop and a right underhand grab. You could also use a left Bong Sao.

Guide your opponent's right arm down as you shift your body to the outside of his guard.

As your opponent's right arm comes down, curl your left hand underneath it. The intention is to grab your opponent's hand so he cannot let go of the knife.

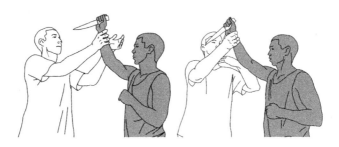

Continue to guide your opponent's arm down until it's horizontal and tight across your body. Your opponent's arm should sit snugly in the crook of your elbow.

Apply the break by pulling your opponent's hand towards you while using your left upper arm to apply opposing pressure on his elbow.

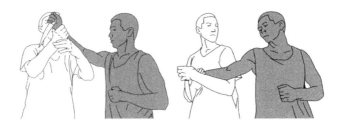

B3 Break

Your opponent attacks with a right straight thrust. Defend with a right chop and a left overhand grab.

Guide your opponent's right hand between your bodies.

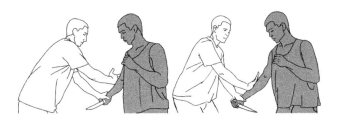

As you do this, use adopt an overhand grip on his right hand with *your* right hand, so he cannot let go of the knife.

Continue to guide your his arm between the two of you until it is horizontal and tight across your body. It should sit snugly in the crook of your elbow.

Apply the break by pulling your opponent's hand towards you whilst using your left upper arm to apply opposing pressure on his elbow.

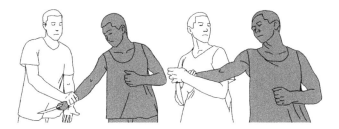

B4 Break

Your opponent attacks with a left straight thrust. Defend with a left Bong Sau and a right overhand grab. You could also use a left chop.

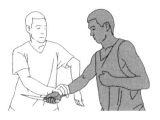

Pull your opponent's right arm across your body as straighten your left arm out perpendicular to his right arm. At this stage, both your elbows should face down. Your opponent's elbow should be on the top of the underside of your elbow.

Grab your opponent's hand with your left hand so he cannot let go of the knife. Apply the break by pulling his hand towards you while using your left upper arm to apply opposing pressure to his elbow.

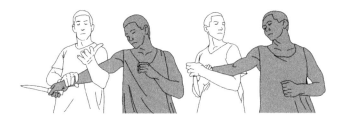

C and D Breaks

The break technique for groups C and D is the same. Your opponent attacks with a right downward thrust. Defend with a left Bong Sau and a right overhand grab. Guide your opponent's arm down as you curl your left arm on top of his elbow.

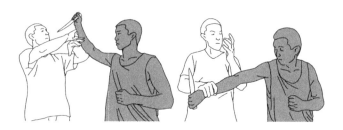

Using a waterfall technique with your left forearm, force your opponent down.

Use your left hand to hold your opponent's shoulder. Place your knee on top of your opponent's elbow and apply downward pressure while pulling up at his wrist and shoulder.

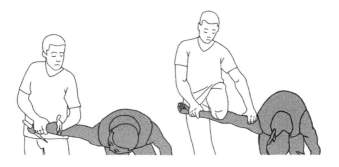

Related Chapters:

- Principles of Self-Defense

UNIVERSALS

Universals are disarming techniques that you can use at any time, no matter what foot you step in with, which block and/or grab you use, or what the angle of attack is.

There are two universal techniques. The following demonstrations show how each of them can be used against the four angles of attack.

Universals 1A

Your opponent attacks with a right downward thrust. Defend with a left Bong Sau and right underhand grab.

Guide your opponent's arm down as you curl your left hand towards you and then overtop of his upper arm. At this point, you may choose to strike him in the face.

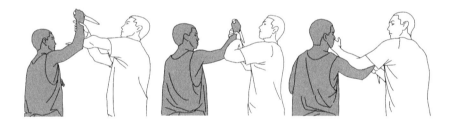

Continue to hook down inside your opponent's guard with your left arm until you grab your own right forearm.

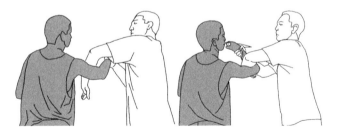

Drive your right elbow into your opponent's face, and then grip the top of the knife with your left hand.

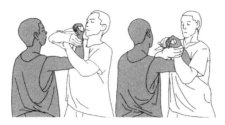

Release your right hand and move it away so you can pry the knife out of your opponent's hand, pulling it toward the outside of his guard.

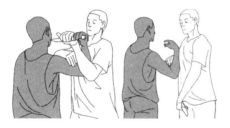

Universals 1B

Your opponent attacks with a left downward thrust. Defend with a left chop and right underhand grip.

Use your left hand to strike your opponent.

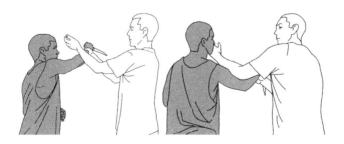

Continue to hook down inside your opponent's guard with your left arm until you grab your own right forearm.

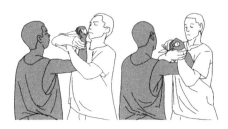

Continue the disarm as previously described.

Universals 1C

Your opponent attacks with a right straight thrust. Defend with a right chop and left overhand grip.

Pass your opponent's right arm between your two bodies. As you do this, adopt an overhand grip on his wrist with your right hand while striking him in the face with your left hand.

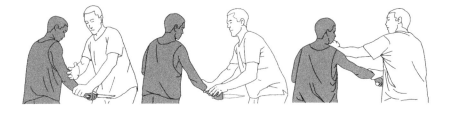

Continue the disarm as previously described. Your right hand can stay in an overhand grip.

Universals 1D

Your opponent attacks with a left straight thrust. Defend with a left chop and right overhand grip.

Use your right hand to raise your opponent's arm a little so you can curl your left arm under.

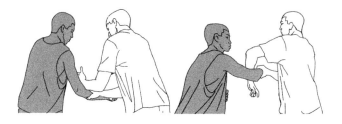

Perform the disarm as previously described.

Universals 2A

Your opponent attacks with a right downward stab. Defend using a left Bong Sau and a right underhand grip. As you guide your opponent's arm down, curl your left arm so it ends up on top of his right elbow.

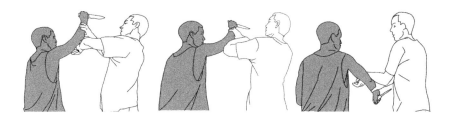

Pass your left hand between your opponent's arm and torso to grab the back of his shoulder. At the same time, move your opponent's arm back with your right hand, so that you stay clear of the knife.

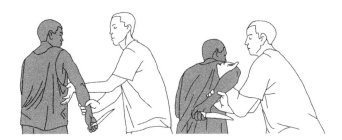

Use your left hand to apply downward pressure on your opponent's shoulder and lock it in place.

Let go of your right hand. Bring it over your opponent's shoulder and grab his right wrist using an underhand grip.

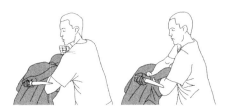

Pull your opponent's wrist towards his right shoulder to apply the lock/break and then take the knife.

Universals 2B

Your opponent attacks with a left downward stab.

Defend with a left chop and right overhand grip.

From there bring your opponent's arm down and perform the disarm as previously described.

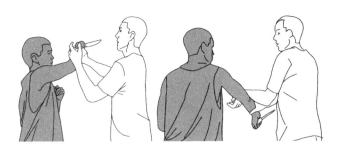

Universals 2C

Your opponent attacks with a right straight thrust. Defend with a right chop and a left overhand grab.

Step to your left so that you're on the outside of your opponent's guard. As you do this, adopt an overhand grip on your opponent's wrist with your right hand.

Once you have a good grip with your left hand, use your right arm to pass between your opponent's arm and body.

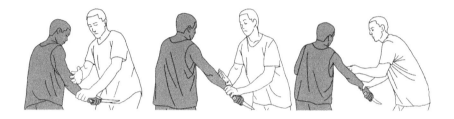

Continue to apply the disarm as previously described.

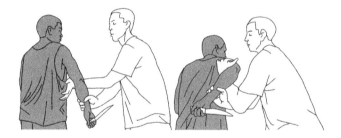

Universals 2D

Your opponent attacks with a left straight thrust. Defend using a left chop and right overhand grab.

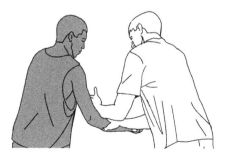

Pass your left arm between your opponent's arm and body, and then continue to apply the disarm as previously described.

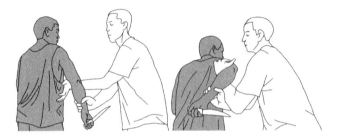

SELF-KILLS

Self-kill techniques are those in which you use the attacker's knife against him while the knife is still in his hand.

This way, you can tell the authorities that you never even touched the knife. He pulled it on you, there was a messy struggle, and he ended up getting hurt.

The label "self-kill" does not mean you have to kill your opponent. A shallow stab in a superficial area will be enough to finish most confrontations.

Self-Kill 1

Your opponent attacks with a right downward stab. Defend using a right Bong Sau and left underhand grab.

Use your right hand to grab your opponent's right wrist with an underhand grip. Facilitate this by bending your opponent's right upper arm to the outside of his guard with your left hand.

Once you have a good grip with your right hand, place your left hand over your opponent's hand so he will not be able to let go of the knife.

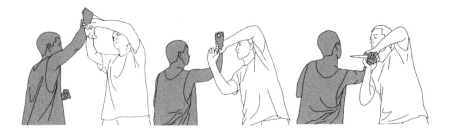

Drive the knife into your opponent's neck. If needed, you can grab the other side of your opponent's neck and pull it into the knife.

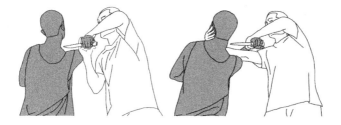

Self-Kill 2

Your opponent attacks with a left downward stab. Defend using a left chop and right underhand grab.

Use your left hand to grab over your opponent's right hand with an overhand grip so that he cannot let go of the knife.

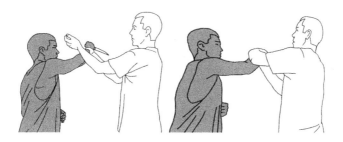

Once you have a good grip, turn the knife towards your opponent and stab him with it.

You can also use your left elbow to apply quick pressure on your opponent's right elbow as a break and/or to soften up his arm.

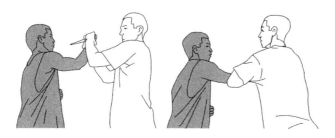

Self-Kill 3

Your opponent attacks with a right straight thrust. Defend using a right chop and left overhand grab.

Use your right hand to grab hold of your opponent's wrist and then move your left hand over his hand. Bend your opponent's wrist down.

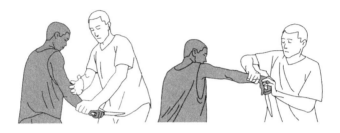

Pull up on your opponent's wrist while pushing his hand down and toward his side.

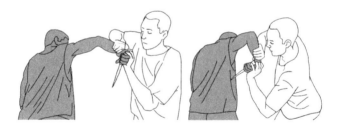

Self-Kill 4

Your opponent attacks with a left straight thrust. Defend using a left chop and right underhand grip.

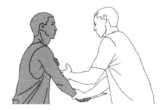

Grab your opponent's hand with your left hand using an overhand grip. Once you have a good grip, move your right hand over the same hand. Your two hands ensure your opponent cannot let go of the knife.

Pull your opponent's arm to the outside of your right shoulder and then fold his wrist back towards him. This will cause his arm to bend so you can slash or stab him.

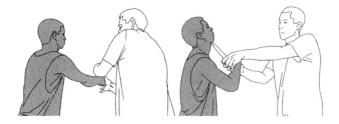

Alternatively, you could also perform a wrist lock.

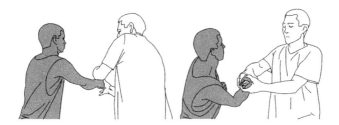

KNIFE FLOW DRILL

It is best if you are at least familiar with all the different disarms described so far before progressing to this knife flow drill.

One person (P1) has a knife and attacks from any angle he chooses. The other person (P2) practices his block/grab defense. P1 then practices countering the block/grab defense. Once free, P1 can then attack again, either from the same angle or a different one.

The countering of the block/grab is the new concept in this drill. P2 should allow P1 to perform the action to begin with. When ready, P2 can start to make things harder by disarming P1 if he is too slow to counter.

There is no set pattern to this drill. The following is just an example of what could happen. When first learning the knife flow drill, you may wish to copy this example, but as you progress, you will learn to instinctively choose the best action in your situation.

P1 attacks with a right downward stab. P2 defends using a left Bong Sau and right underhand grip.

P2 curls his left forearm underneath and then on top of P1's arm, and then grabs his knife-wielding hand.

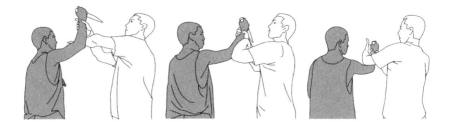

P1 uses his left hand to push on P2's elbow and free his hand.

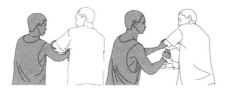

P1 attacks with a left downward stab. P2 defends with a left chop and right underhand grab. P2 uses his left hand to grab P1's thumb and then twists it to the outside of P1's guard.

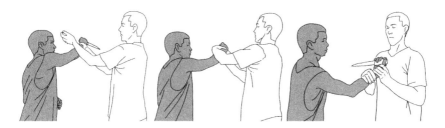

P1 pushes up on P2's right wrist to free his hand. P1 attacks with a right straight thrust. P2 defends with a right chop and left underhand grab.

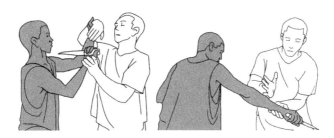

P2 uses his right hand to grab P1's right hand and bends his wrist down. P2 then twists P1's arm clockwise, so that his elbow is facing up.

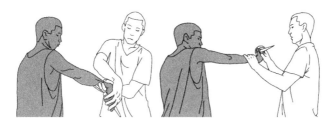

P1 uses his left hand to push up on P2's wrist to free his hand. P1 attacks with a left straight thrust. P2 defends with a left chop and right underhand grab.

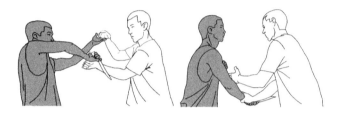

P2 grabs P1's hand with his left hand and applies a wrist lock by twisting P1's arm to the outside of his guard.

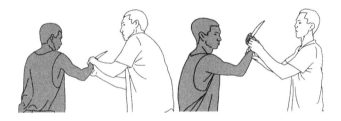

Before the lock is applied, P1 pushes up on P2's right hand to release the grip.

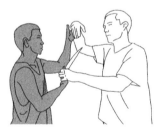

The rest of this demonstration shows some alternative flows focusing on the first strike—that is, a downward right stab. This same idea can be applied to any strike/defense/counter. It's presented here just to give you an idea of how you can adapt this drill in training.

P1 attacks with a right downward strike again. P2 defends with a left Bong Sau and right overhand grip. P2 uses his right hand to grab P1's right thumb and begins to bring it down.

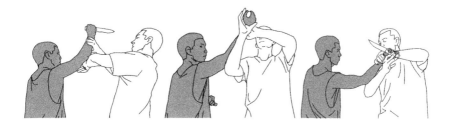

P1 hits down on his own right arm at the crook of his elbow to escape the hold.

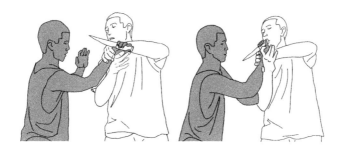

Note: If P2 uses a proper grip and continues into Self Kill 1, P1 will probably not be able to do this reversal.

P1 attacks with a right downward strike again. P2 defends with a left Bong Sau and right overhand grip. P2 curls his left forearm underneath and then on top of P1's arm, and then grabs his knife-wielding hand.

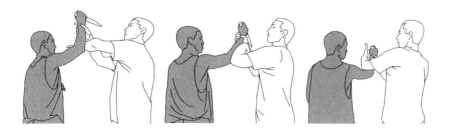

P1 uses his left hand to push on P2's elbow to free his hand.

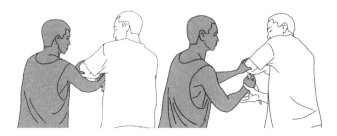

P2 then uses his left hand to grab P2's left arm and applies an arm break.

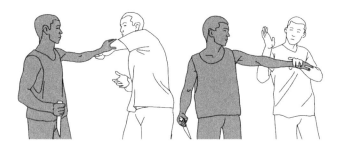

P1 attacks with a right downward strike again and P2 catches P1's wrist with his right hand.

P2 brings his right hand over P1's right arm to apply a lock.

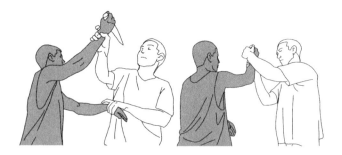

P1 pushes up at P2's left wrist to release his arm.

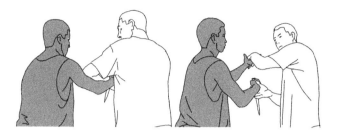

This completes the knife flow drill demonstration. As you may real-
ize, it has infinite variations.

Related Chapters:

- Defense

BONUS CHAPTERS

The following bonus chapters are direct excerpts from *The Self-Defense Handbook* by Sam Fury.

www.SFNonfictionBooks.com/Self-Defense-Handbook

IMPROVISED WEAPONS

When running isn't an option, and you have the opportunity to get one, use a weapon.

If you can hit with, thrust, throw, spray, or hide behind something, it's a potential improvised weapon. That covers almost any object, though some are better than others.

A good improvised weapon is one that you can carry around without suspicion—that is, one a police officer would not take off you in the street. Examples of such weapons are:

- An umbrella
- A pen
- Hairspray and a lighter (for a makeshift flamethrower)

There are four types of improvised weapons that are the best to use for self-defense:

- Knives
- Clubs
- Shields
- Projectiles

When training with improvised weapons, choose things you routinely carry around, like an umbrella, a pen, or trade tools.

The generic grip for any weapon is to hold it firmly in your fist, but not so tightly that doing so causes fatigue. Put your legs in an aggressive ready stance.

Knives

Knives are one-handed thrusting objects. Besides an actual knife, you could use a bottle, scissors, a rolled-up magazine, etc.

Hold the knife in your strong hand and use a weak lead.

Position your knife hand down and back at your waist. Use your lead hand to guard.

Thrust straight out at your opponent's abdomen and bring your arm straight back

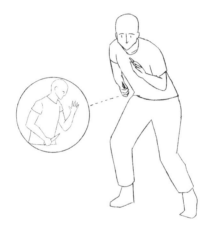

Clubs

A club can be any solid object that is too big to be a knife, but not so big that it's cumbersome. A metal pipe, a baseball bat, a walking stick, etc., are all good clubs.

Hold your club in both hands, up behind your shoulder. Alternatively, hold it in one hand and use the other as a guard.

Strike straight down into your opponent's head, and/or thrust the club into his face or gut. You can also strike his knee, which is a less damaging target, but will still put him out of commission.

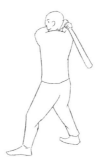

Shields

Anything you can hide behind or use as an obstacle—a chair, a door, a wall, a backpack, etc.— makes a good shield.

If you can pick it up, use it to block and thrust. If it's an immovable object, ram your opponent's head into it.

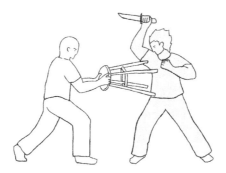

Projectiles

A projectile is anything you can throw or spray that isn't better used some other way, such as an ashtray, deodorant, hot liquid, or dirt.

Tactical Pen

A tactical pen is a good example of a knife weapon that you can carry around without suspicion. The best type of tactical pen for self-defense is one that you'll carry. Any simple stainless-steel pen will work, but ideally, you'll choose one that:

- Is refillable
- Writes well (you like it)
- Has a clip
- Has a flat top (that won't stab you)
- Is easy to replace/inexpensive
- Can pass as a normal pen (to get through security)

Most of the tactical pens on the market do not fill these requirements, especially the last one. Those that do include:

- Zebra 701
- Zebra 402
- Parker Jotter
- Fisher Space Military Pen (this one is a little more expensive, but still under $20)

Clip your tactical pen somewhere on your body that is easy to access with your dominant hand, such as your front pants pocket on your dominant side. Put it in the same place every time and practice deploying it, so doing so becomes second nature.

When you grab the pen, hold it in an icepick grip, with your thumb on top.

Every time you initially grab the pen, including to write something or to put it away, use this grip.

Grab the pen and thrust it straight into your opponent in one swift movement. A cardboard box makes a good target when training.

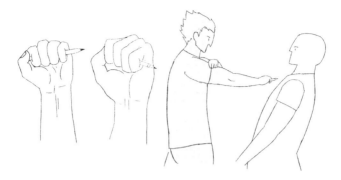

You can strike from almost any angle. Thrust the pen into any target area to help you escape.

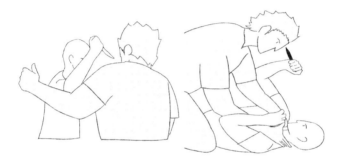

Sap

Anything heavy in a sock makes a good improvised sap. You can use coins, a billiard ball, a soda can, or a rock.

Another way to make one is to tie a metal nut (or something similar) to a piece of cord, such as a shoelace.

A piece of material about the size of a tea towel (or t-shirt) with a small weighted object (like a handful of coins) in it also works.

- Put the object in the center of the material.
- Fold the material diagonally in half over the object.
- Roll up the material from the point to the base.

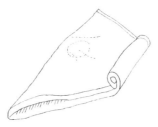

Hold both ends so the object in the middle is now the striking end.
Use it like a club—that is, make vertical strikes to your opponent's
head. You can also uppercut.

WEAPON VS WEAPON

If you're going to fight someone with a weapon, getting your own weapon will give you the best chance of success.

In addition to the following information, review the Improvised Weapons chapter.

Your opponent's hand makes a good secondary target if it's closer than his head.

When using a knife, use timing, footwork, and feints. Wait for your opponent to strike and then close in before he can recover. You can use a feint to time his strike.

If you have a club, use the overhead strike straight down along the central line. If your opponent uses an angled attack, your straight overhead will win. When you both use the overhead strike, the strike that hits its target first will succeed.

If your opponent's strike is going to beat yours, parry it. As his strike comes in, tap the top of your weapon on his to deflect it. Immediately return your club to the center line to finish your strike.

When you hold a longer weapon, keep the advantage of distance. Use footwork, overhead strikes, and thrusts.

Related Chapters:

- Improvised Weapons

THANKS FOR READING

Dear reader,

Thank you for reading *Practical Escrima Knife Defense.*

If you enjoyed this book, please leave a review where you bought it. It helps more than most people think.

Don't forget your FREE book chapters!

You will also be among the first to know of FREE review copies, discount offers, bonus content, and more.

Go to:

https://offers.SFNonfictionBooks.com/Free-Chapters

Thanks again for your support.

REFERENCES

Abenir, F. (2014). *Eskrima Street Defense: Practical Techniques for Dangerous Situations*. Tambuli Media.

Anderson, D. (2013). *De-Fanging The Snake: A Guide To Modern Arnis Disarms*. CreateSpace Independent Publishing Platform.

Anderson, D. (2013). *Filipino Martial Arts - The Core Basics, Structure, & Essentials*. CreateSpace Independent Publishing Platform.

Anderson, D. (2014). *Trankada: The Joint Locking Techniques & Tapi-Tapi of Modern Arnis*. CreateSpace Independent Publishing Platform.

Buot, S. (2015). *Balintawak Eskrima*. Allegro Editions.

Diega, A. Ricketts, C. (2002). *The Secrets of Kalis Ilustrisimo: The Filipino Fighting Art Explained*. Tuttle Publishing.

Godhania, K. (2012). *Eskrima: Filipino Martial Art*. Crowood.

Gould, D. (2016). *Lameco Eskrima: The Legacy of Edgar G. Sulite*. Tambuli Media.

Medina, D. (2014). *The Secret Art of Derobio Escrima: Martial Art of the Philippines*. Tambuli Media.

Paman, J. (2007). *Arnis Self-Defense: Stick, Blade, and Empty-Hand Combat Techniques of the Philippines*. Blue Snake Books.

Pentecost, D. (2016). *Put 'Em Down. Take 'Em Out!: Knife Fighting Techniques From Folsom Prison*. Allegro Editions.

Presas, R. (1983). *Modern Arnis: The Filipino Art of Stick Fighting*. Black Belt Communications.

Preto, L. (2016). *Multiple opponent combat: 10 lesson program with one handed weapons*. CreateSpace Independent Publishing Platform.

Wiley, M. (2011). *Secrets of Cabales Serrada Escrima*. Tuttle Publishing.

Wiley, M. (2015). *Mastering Eskrima Disarms*. Tambuli Media.

AUTHOR RECOMMENDATIONS

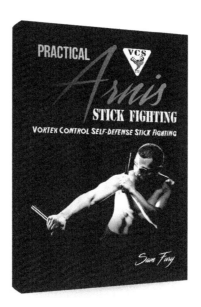

Teach Yourself Stick Fighting for Self-Defense

Teach yourself *Practical Arnis Stick Fighting* today, because the traditional
stuff doesn't work on the streets.

Get it now.

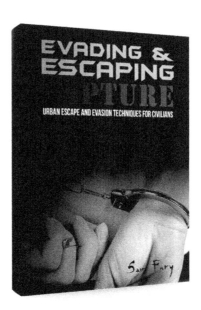

Teach Yourself Escape and Evasion Tactics

Discover the skills you need to evade and escape capture, because you never know when they will save your life.

Get it now.

www.SFNonfictionBooks.com/Evading-Escaping-Capture

ABOUT SAM FURY

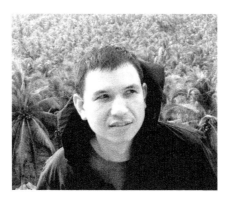

Sam Fury has had a passion for survival, evasion, resistance, and escape (SERE) training since he was a young boy growing up in Australia.

This led him to years of training and career experience in related subjects, including martial arts, military training, survival skills, outdoor sports, and sustainable living.

These days, Sam spends his time refining existing skills, gaining new skills, and sharing what he learns via the Survival Fitness Plan website.

www.SurvivalFitnessPlan.com

amazon.com/author/samfury

goodreads.com/SamFury

facebook.com/AuthorSamFury

instagram.com/AuthorSamFury

youtube.com/SurvivalFitnessPlan

Printed in Great Britain
by Amazon